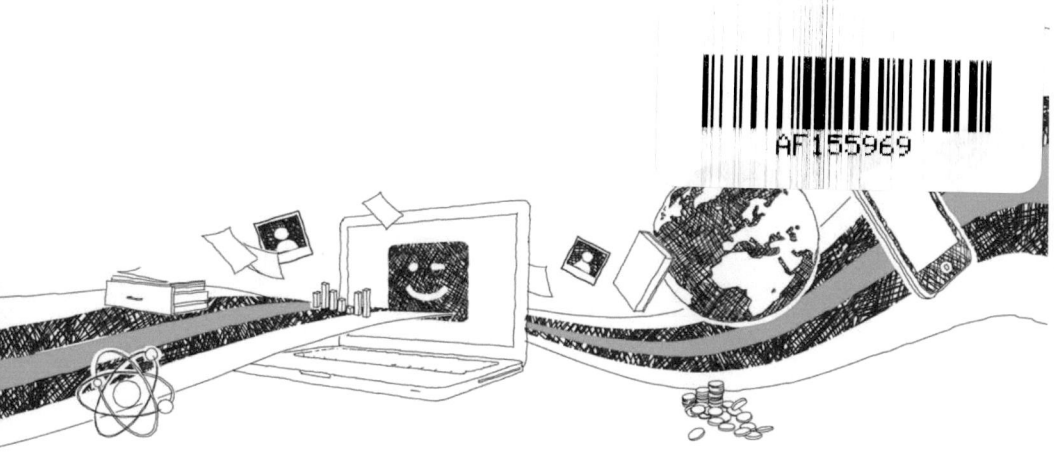
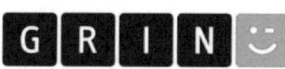

Deanna Di Gregorio

Strategies to Improve the Canadian Healthcare System

GRIN Publishing

Bibliographic information published by the German National Library:

The German National Library lists this publication in the National Bibliography; detailed bibliographic data are available on the Internet at http://dnb.dnb.de .

Imprint:

Copyright © 2010 GRIN Verlag GmbH
Print and binding: Books on Demand GmbH, Norderstedt Germany
ISBN: 978-3-640-80054-4

This book at GRIN:

http://www.grin.com/en/e-book/164839/strategies-to-improve-the-canadian-healthcare-system

GRIN - Your knowledge has value

Since its foundation in 1998, GRIN has specialized in publishing academic texts by students, college teachers and other academics as e-book and printed book. The website www.grin.com is an ideal platform for presenting term papers, final papers, scientific essays, dissertations and specialist books.

Visit us on the internet:

http://www.grin.com/

http://www.facebook.com/grincom

http://www.twitter.com/grin_com

Recommendations for Strategies to Improve the Canadian Healthcare System

Deanna Di Gregorio

Health Science 4410A

December 6, 2010

Pages: 15

Table of Contents

Introduction

Canadian Healthcare: A Brief Overview

Canada's universal healthcare system, frequently referred to as "Medicare," was introduced in 1962 solely to the province of Saskatchewan by premier, Tommy Douglas. In 1964, Emmet Hall published the Hall Commission, which recommended that all provinces and territories adopt a universal healthcare program similar to Saskatchewan. By 1972, all provinces and territories had established universal health coverage programs, providing medically necessary services to all Canadians. The Canada Health Act of 1984 was enacted with the mandate "to protect, promote and restore the physical and mental well-being of residents of Canada and to facilitate reasonable access to health services without financial or other barriers" (L. Hughes-Marsh, personal communication, September 20, 2010). The Act has five principles: (1) public administration, healthcare must be administered by the provinces on a non-profit basis by public authority; (2) comprehensiveness, health insurance plans must cover all medically necessary services; (3) universality, all insured residents are able to access public healthcare services; (4) portability, provinces are required to cover citizens when they are temporarily absent from their home province; and (5) accessibility, all insured citizens have reasonable access to insured services (Canadian Health Care, 2004). The aforementioned policies and principles have assisted in creating the universal, *glorious and free* healthcare system that historically Canadians have been so proud to adopt as part of their identity.

The 2010 Report Card however, suggests that this attitude is shifting. When compared with six other developed nations on the performance of their healthcare systems, Canada ranked sixth, only placing ahead of the United States, the one country that does not have universal healthcare. Factors measured include: quality of care, access, efficiency, equity and health outcomes (L. Hughes-Marsh, personal communication, September 20, 2010). These findings provide evidence that Canadians no longer hold the same value for their once glorified, universal

healthcare system. Instead, the system receives an abundance of criticism for its inability to

provide quality care to all citizens and is thus currently facing many challenges and structural

reforms. This report will outline three recommendations to improve the current Canadian

healthcare system: going lean in healthcare, establishing universal prescription drug coverage

programs and incorporating virtual health practices into the Canadian healthcare system. Since

healthcare is mandated on a provincial level, the aforementioned recommendations will be

primarily targeted to Ontario. Once these recommendations have successfully been adopted in

Ontario, the federal government can encourage other provinces and territories to adopt similar

practices.

Recommendation One

Going Lean in Healthcare

Lean thinking was developed at Toyota Manufacturing plants in Japan and involves

eliminating waste "so that all work adds value and serve's the customer's needs" (Innovation

Series 2005: Going Lean in Health Care, 2005). At Toyota Manufacturing plants, management

looked for ways to eliminate waste (or *muda* in Japanese) in the current system of vehicle

production. Lean thinking involves distinguishing value-added from non-value-added steps,

removing the seven types of *muda* (Appendix A); simply stated it is striving for perfection, so

that all steps add value to the process. Although healthcare and the manufacturing of vehicles

seem very different on the surface, the end result of providing value to the customer, in this case

the patient, is the same. Both focus on zero defects through quality, safety, cost and customer

and employee satisfaction. Striving for perfection in healthcare is necessary to avoid injuries. In

the United States, while working at 99.9% levels of quality, approximately 500 incorrect surgeries are performed each week (D. Lee, personal communication, October 8, 2009). This

statistic emphasizes the importance of striving for zero defects and going lean.

Through the adoption of lean thinking, hospitals can develop a strategy, similar to that of

Virginia Mason Hospital and Medical Center in the United States (Appendix B), which places the

patient first. Here, *kaizen*, continuous improvement of processes, is an important part of the

corporate culture. Studies have shown that when applied carefully, lean thinking can have a

tremendous impact on the productivity, cost and quality of services provided by an organization

(Innovative Series: 2005, Going Lean in Healthcare, 2005). When hospitals focus on the

specified needs of the patient, he or she is better able to flow through the system without waits or

delays, thereby creating a more efficient process. Through value stream mapping, hospitals

identify specific activities necessary to deliver services to the patient and eliminate *muda*.

One such example is the 5-S (Sort, Simplify, Standardize, Sweep and Self-Discipline)

method of organizing workspaces. The method embraces the philosophy that all items have a

place, and that they all should be in that place, clean and ready to use for the next worker

(D. Lee, personal communication, October 8, 2009). This simple organizational philosophy can

significantly increase the productivity of a workplace through neatly arranging and appropriately

labeling articles so that workers can easily locate specific items (Appendix C). The differences

with respect to the organization of the workbenches in Figures 2 and 3 of Appendix C are

shocking. In Figure 3, all medical items are neatly placed and labeled in their designated spot,

while in Figure 2 everything is cluttered; an accident waiting to happen.

Another important component of lean thinking, involves establishing standard work.

Taiichi Ohno, Vice President of Toyota Motor Corporation states that, "Where there is no

standard, there can be no *kaizen*" (D. Lee, personal communication, October 8, 2009). Standard

work is the safest, most efficient way to perform a particular task and yields the highest quality result. The four steps comprising standard work include observing the work, analyzing and

identifying *muda*, eliminating *muda* by trying out the process and creating a new standard for the

work cycle. Similar to all lean practices standard work is continuously improved, hence *kaizen*.

Lean healthcare has the ability to improve the quality of care, safety of workplaces and

patient and employee satisfaction, while improving productivity and thereby reducing costs. It

puts patient satisfaction first and focuses on meeting his or her needs, which should be the

standard when delivering care. If the patient is not satisfied, the operation, procedure or service

was not successful. Workplaces involved in the delivery of healthcare services must adopt lean

thinking strategies, so that they can be incorporated into the organization's corporate culture. As

with implementing any new strategy or program, initially resistance from staff will exist. Lean

thinking challenges all employees to work together, emanating the lean philosophy throughout

the entire organization. With the participation of all healthcare staff and administration, the

waste in the current Canadian system can continue to be identified and eliminated, thereby

positively influencing, costs, quality, productivity and the delivery of medical services in a timely

manner.

Recommendation Two

Universal Prescription Drug Coverage

Throughout Canada a nationwide, universal prescription drug program does not exist.

The Ontario Drug Benefit (ODB) program allows select populations to receive prescription drug

coverage. This includes those who are: over the age of 65, long-term care home residents,

residents of Homes for Special Care, recipients of services through the Home Care program and

registered in the Trillium Drug Program. In contrast, a large proportion of the provincial

population who are ineligible for the ODB program have two options: to either use a private

insurance plan or pay out of pocket (Ontario Ministry of Health and Long Term Care, 2009).

From a global perspective, Sweden has one of the largest aging populations in the world, yet has one of the highest life expectancies. When compared with Canada, Sweden has a greater life expectancy, lower infant mortality rate and spends both less per capita and a lower percentage of their GDP on healthcare (World Health Organization, 2008). Similar to Canada, Sweden has a universal healthcare system, however, unlike Canada, they provide prescription drug coverage to their citizens.

The state, county councils and patients finance prescription drugs in Sweden. Since the county councils oversee healthcare, they are responsible for covering the cost of all inpatient medicines. Taxes are levied to finance such benefits. The outpatient prescription drug program applies to all legal residents of Sweden; the county councils receive grants from the government, which are allocated toward this. In 2005, the state paid approximately 2.2 billion Euros, which was more than sufficient to cover the cost. Although the state and county councils pay for a large proportion of outpatient medicine, patients also contribute. However, the policy does not allow citizens to spend more than 200 Euro in a 12-month period on prescription drugs. On average, patients cover approximately 21% of the cost associated with outpatient medicine. All costs for children under the age of eighteen in an individual family are grouped together. Persons who cannot afford to spend the 200 Euro maximum can apply to have costs subsidized. The county councils have committees that assess all individuals and families on a case-by-case basis (Pharmaceutical Benefits Board, 2007). In Ontario, the Local Health Integration Networks (LHINs) would oversee this process. The program is structured around the usage of more cost efficient generic rather than brand name drugs. However, if a patient specifies that he or she would like the brand name drug, they are required to pay the cost difference between the two products. Cost negotiations and decisions regarding which drugs should be subsidized, are made by the Pharmaceutical Benefits Board, a division of the county councils (Pharmaceutical Benefits

Board, 2007). In 2008, Sweden spent approximately $3 billion (CAD) on outpatient prescription drugs, while Ontario spent $3.6 billion (CAD) with the ODB program. Sweden managed to spend less on 9 million people, than Ontario did on 3 million (D. Lee, personal communication, November 26, 2009).

Implementing this program in Ontario will result in resistance from seniors, private insurance companies and pharmacies. In order to combat this resistance, the deductible for senior citizens could be increased, private insurance companies could continue to operate for those individuals seeking brand name drugs, and pharmacists could enjoy the perks of working for the government, for example job security, which is not present in private organizations. Although limitations and barriers to entry in Ontario do exist, the results and benefits observed in Sweden have the potential to better both the Ontario and Canadian healthcare systems through the incorporation of a universal outpatient prescription drug coverage program.

Recommendation Three

Incorporating Virtual Health Practices

Current physician shortages and inefficiencies in healthcare settings are making it difficult for patients to access healthcare services in a timely manner. A solution that some medical practices are turning to involves using the Internet as a mode of communication. The Virtual Practice, currently a pilot project at Massachusetts General Hospital, consists of an electronic medical record (EMR) and Patient Portal, which allow physicians to communicate with and provide care to patients, regardless of distance. The EMR contains the patient's clinical data and can be shared amongst physicians, promoting communication and guaranteeing continuity of care. The Patient Portal is an online system where the patient can communicate with the practice and physician just as they would at the physician's office; appointments, prescription refills and the review of test results can all be accomplished through the portal. Patients given a secure username and password are able to access the portal at any computer via the Internet (Dixon &

Perrotti, 2008).

Virtual Practice is not a replacement for the doctor-patient relationship, but creates a more

efficient means of healthcare delivery. Comprised of three components, the medical

advancement uses videoconferencing to deliver care and manage disease. The three components

are: (1) asynchronous consultation with the provider team, guides the patient through scripted

templates simulating a doctor's visit, gathering information in an easy to interpret form for the

provider; (2) synchronous communication with the provider, allows the physician to evaluate the

patient when an office visit is not required; and (3) remote physiologic monitoring, which helps

the physician and patient collaborate in the management of chronic illness and disease, while

decreasing the burden of unnecessary visits to the practice (Dixon & Perrotti, 2008).

This technological advancement has the ability to bridge gaps in the current Canadian healthcare

system. Canada has one of the worst rural-urban gaps in healthcare, with urban populations

being significantly healthier than their rural counterparts (C. Brown, personal communication,

September 21, 2010). Studies have shown that rural populations have both lower functional and

self-rated health when compared to urban residents (Rural and Small Town Canada Analysis

Bulletin, 2004). The successful implementation of this technology can positively influence and

reduce this gap, connecting rural patients who may not have a family or local physician, as well

as, easing a doctor's ability to provide check-ups and monitor the patient's health. If further

consultation is required, the physician can request that the patient book an in-office appointment,

where a more detailed analysis can be conducted (Dixon & Perrotti, 2008).

Studies have shown patients are satisfied with the virtual visit, but when given a choice,

they prefer the in-person consultation with the physician (Dixon & Perrotti, 2008). The

implementation of this technology will likely receive patient resistance at first, but as the practice grows in popularity, the negative attitude will subside. It is worth noting that although

physicians are limited in terms of physical examinations that they are able to conduct, their

ability to take patient history and diagnose certain conditions was not significantly different

between teleconferencing and in office visits (Dixon & Perrotti, 2008). Additionally the Virtual

Practice is limited in its ability to become commonplace in primary care settings because large

organizational and financial support must be present. However, given the vast geography of

Canada, the Virtual Practice offers great prospect in ensuring that the healthcare system lives up

to the five principles of the Canada Health Act, by positively influencing the universality and

accessibility of healthcare services.

Conclusion

Though the above three initiatives are very different with respect to their specific focus,

they all share the potential to improve the Canadian healthcare system. Given the large amount

of critique that healthcare receives for wasted initiatives, a solution is the adoption of lean

thinking, so that such waste in the current system can be identified and eliminated, thereby

creating a more efficient and productive system and thus an overall better patient experience.

One area of such waste is the provincial expense accumulated on providing drugs to a limited

proportion of the population. Adopting a universal prescription drug program similar to Sweden

can provide all Canadians with access to affordable prescription drugs and lower the expense.

Another weakness in the Canadian healthcare system relates to discrepancies between rural and

urban settings, with the former needing much improvement. This paper promotes the initiation of

the Virtual Practice, which has the potential to reduce gaps in the current system by bringing

physicians and patients together, wherever they are, no matter the distance between them.

Currently the Canadian healthcare system is receiving numerous criticisms for its waste,

prescription drug coverage and gaps in access to healthcare. These important issues question whether or not the current delivery of services reflects the principles of the Canada Health Act,

specifically universality and accessibility. The aforementioned strategies: lean thinking,

developing a universal prescription drug coverage program and incorporating virtual practices

will help the Canadian healthcare system live up to all five principles of the Canada Health Act.

Through the adoption of these recommendations Canadians can regain their *glorious and free*

universal healthcare system, a system that they should be proud to be a part of.

References

Brown, C. (2010, September 21). Personal communication.

Canadian Health Care. (2004). Canada Health Act. Retrieved from
http://www.canadian-healthcare.org/page2.html

Dixon, R.F., & Perrotti, R. (Ed.). (2008). *The virtual practice: tomorrow's medicine, today*.
Boston, MA, USA

Innovation Series 2005: Going lean in health care. (2005). Cambridge, MA: Institute for
Healthcare Improvement.

Health Canada, (2010). *Canada's health care system (Medicare)* Retrieved November 2,
2010, from http://www.hc-sc.gc.ca/hcs-sss/medi-assur/index-eng.php

Health Canada, (2004). *Federal public drug benefit programs* Retrieved November 2, 2010,
from http://www.hc-sc.gc.ca/hcs-sss/pharma/acces/fedprog-eng.php

Health Canada, (2009). *Provincial/territorial role in health* Retrieved November 2, 2010,
from http://www.hc-sc.gc.ca/hcs-sss/delivery-prestation/ptrole/index-eng.php

Hughes-Marsh, L. (2010, September 20). Personal communication.

Lee, D. (2009, October 8). Personal communication.

Lee, D. (2009, November 26). Personal communication.

Ontario Ministry of Health and Long-Term Care, (2009). *Ontario drug benefit : the program*
Retrieved November 4, 2010, from
http://www.health.gov.on.ca/english/public/pub/drugs/odb.html

Pharmaceutical Benefits Board. (2007). The Swedish Pharmaceutical Reimbursement
System. Retrieved November 5, 2010, from
http://www.tlv.se/Upload/English/ENG-swe-pharma-reimbursement-system.pdf

Rural and Small Town Canada Analysis Bulletin. (2004). Health status and behaviours of
Canada's youth: a rural-urban comparison. Retrieved from
http://dsp-psd.pwgsc.gc.ca/Collection/Statcan/21-006-X/21-006-XIE2003003.pdf

Sweden. Ministry of Health and Social Affairs. (2004) *Health and medical care policy*.
Retrieved November 6, 2010, from http://www.sweden.gov.se/sb/d/2950

World Health Organization. (2008). *Sweden: Statistics*. Retrieved November 15, 2010, from
http://www.who.int/countries/swe/en/

Appendix A

Table 1: The Seven Types of Muda According to Lean Thinking

Waste Type	Definition
Motion	Unnecessary movement or movement that does not add value
Defects	Waste related to costs for inspection of defects in materials and processes, customer complaints and repairs
Transportation	Transferring, picking up, setting down and otherwise moving unnecessary items
Inventory	Having more on hand that what is needed and used
Overproduction	Producing what is unnecessary, when it is unnecessary and in unnecessary amounts
Time	Time wasted waiting for people or services to be provided and when your people, processes and machines are idle
Processing	Unnecessary processes and operations traditionally accepted as necessary

(D. Lee, personal communication, October 8, 2009)

Appendix B

Figure 1: Virgin Mason's Strategic Plan for the Delivery of Healthcare Services

(D. Lee, personal communication, October 8, 2009)

Figure 6. The Virginia Mason Medical Center Strategic Plan

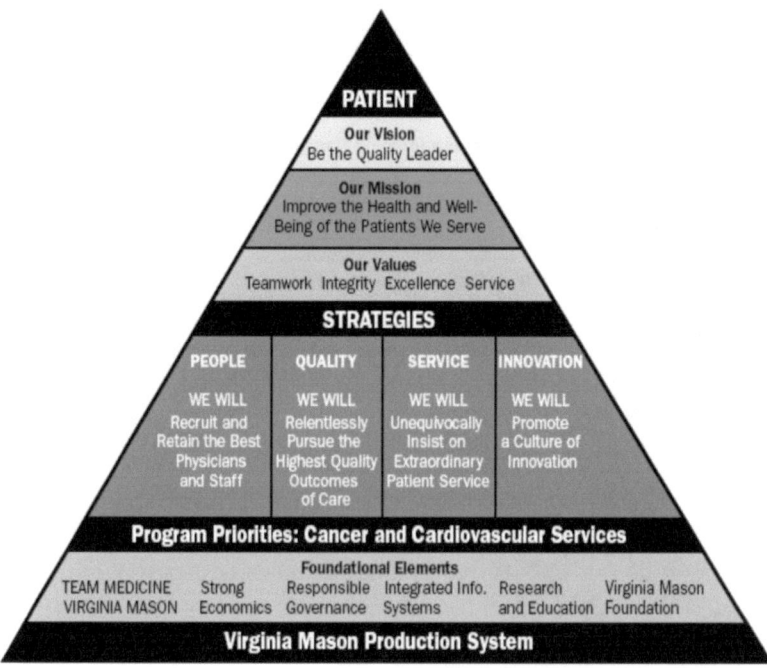

Source: Virginia Mason Medical Center

(D. Lee, personal communication, October 8, 2009)

Appendix C

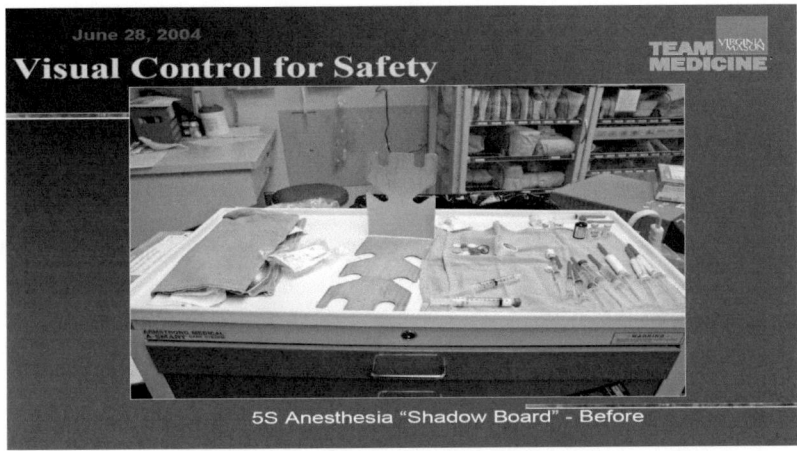

Figure 2: Anesthesia Shadow Board Before 5S

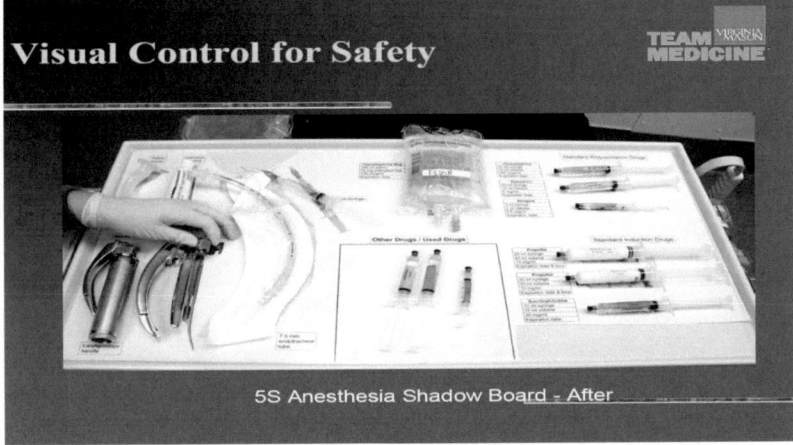

Figure 3: Anesthesia Shadow Board After 5S

(D. Lee, personal communication, October 8, 2009)